MW00761382

*In appreciation
for your help and*

COMPASSIONATE VEGETARIANS

sincere concern.

Holly

AN ILLUSTRATED JOURNEY

COMPASSIONATE VEGETARIANS

An Illustrated Journey

HOLLY HARLAYNE ROBERTS

ANJELI PRESS, INC.

COMPASSIONATE VEGETARIANS

AN ILLUSTRATED JOURNEY

Written and Illustrated by
Holly Harlayne Roberts, D.O., Ph.D.

Published by
Anjeli Press
www.AnjeliPress.com

ISBN 0-9754844-4-3

In appreciation to Heather Victoria Roberts
for her origami artwork.

Printed in the United States
by Lightning Source
Distributed by Ingram Distributors

Dedicated to Edgar Kupfer-Koberwitz

Edgar Kupfer-Koberwitz (1906–) scrawled the following letter on scraps of paper with pieces of pencil while confined to a hospital barracks in Concentration Camp Dachau. This was a time when death grasped, day by day, his people in that camp. They lost twelve thousand within four and a half months. For three years, Edgar Kupfer hid these writings.

I eat no animals, because I don't want to live off the suffering and death of other creatures—I suffered so much myself, that I can feel other creatures' suffering, by virtue of my own.

I am so glad when nobody harms me; so why should I harm others or have them harmed? I am so glad not to be injured or killed; so why should I injure or kill other creatures or have them injured or killed for my sake. Isn't it only natural that I don't want anything to happen to other creatures that I don't want happening to myself?

I want to live in a more beautiful world, a world with higher, more blissful rules, with a divine rule for all future: Love for all Creation.[1]

[1] Kupfer-Koberwitz, Edgar, Papers, *Dachau Diaries*, Special Collections Research Center, University of Chicago Library. From the

My motivation in writing this book has been to express the deeply sensitive sentiments shared by millions of individuals, over countless generations, who have chosen to live without taking the lives of other beings to sustain their own existences.

It has always seemed quite unfortunate to me that the term *vegetarian* has been chosen to describe the lifestyles of such empathetic, idealist, and self-sacrificing individuals—individuals who could not even dream of taking the life of another being merely to consume its flesh.

I believe a more appropriate term for such individuals might have been: *empathetic dieters, thoughtful sustainers, merciful consumers, followers of nonviolence,* or *compassionate vegetarians.*

The term *compassionate vegetarians* expresses the reality that these individuals have chosen to live such lifestyles to spare billions of weaker beings from suffering the ravages of tortured existences and untimely, tragic deaths.

I hope this book conveys the meaningful, sensitive, and empathetic values of those who might best be described as *compassionate vegetarians.*

translation of Ruth Mossner, who placed her translation in the public domain.

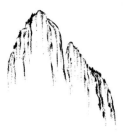

Vegetarians do not follow a diet—
They follow a way of life.

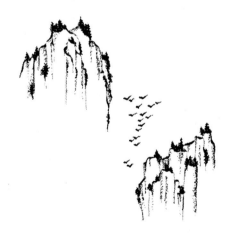

Vegetarians seek to live
showing mercy to all beings.

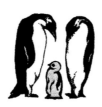

Compassionate
Vegetarians
seek
to live
without
abundance.

Their lives
are
simple,
humble,
and
peaceful.

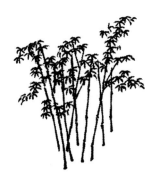

Vegetarians believe in the sanctity of life—
all life.

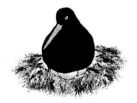

Vegetarians believe
that
any being
that longs to protect
its young

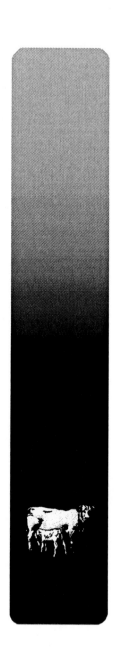

is a being who
feels fear,
compassion,
and love.

Vegetarians seek to live in peace
with all other beings
with whom they share
this blessed planet.

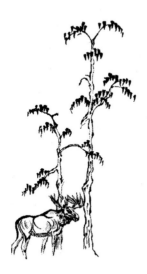

Vegetarians seek
to sustain
their existence
on those
foods,
the consumption
of which,
does not inflict
pain
and suffering
on any other
being.

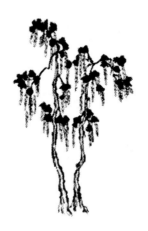

Vegetarians believe that all created beings
love life.

Vegetarians believe
that kindness
should not be
restricted
solely to those
within
specific species.

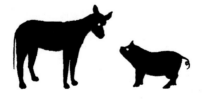

Vegetarians believe
that even the humblest of beings
possesses a soul.

Many who wish to share the blessings of life with all beings—become vegetarian.

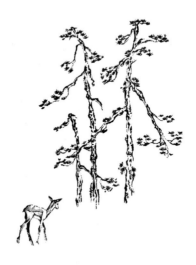

Vegetarians view their brief sojurn on
earth as a chance to share kindness
with—

the humble,
the small,
and the weak.

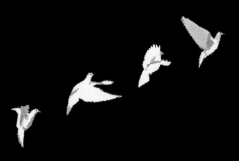

Vegetarians
believe
that if
humankind
seeks to secure peace
on our
planet
we must
first secure
peace
for all
weaker
beings.

Vegetarians feel compassion
for all
suffering beings—
excluding none.

Vegetarians
do
not
seek
to
assert
power
and
dominance
over
weak,
vulnerable
creatures.

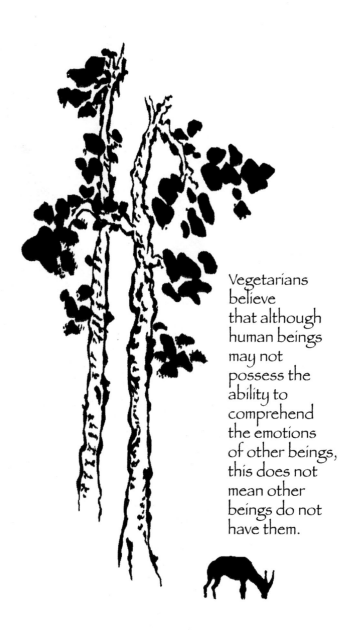

Vegetarians
believe
that although
human beings
may not
possess the
ability to
comprehend
the emotions
of other beings,
this does not
mean other
beings do not
have them.

Vegetarians
recognize
that the desire
to live
without taking
life from others
cannot be easily taught—
It is an emotion
that evolves
within
the depths
of one's soul.

Vegetarians value the varying gifts
of all people,
all creatures,
and, indeed,
all creation.

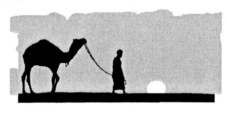

Although vegetarians may not gain
the acceptance of others,

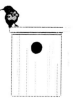

they live
guided by their own
sense of values.

Vegetarians believe that all beings
harbor longings, dreams, and hopes.

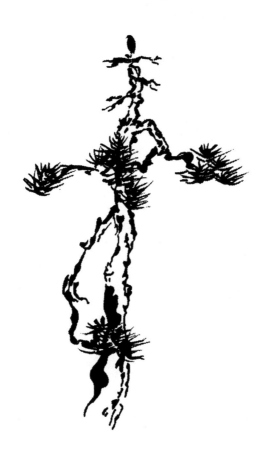

Vegetarians
never find
their lifestyle
a chore.

To them,
it is a privilege.

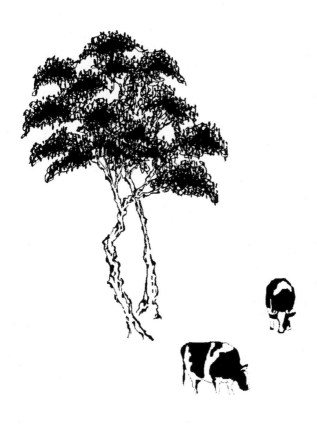

Vegetarians value the teachings
of Saint Francis of Assisi—

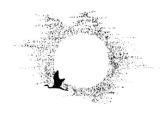

love for all people,
concern for all creatures,
and appreciation for all creation.

Vegetarians hope that, someday,
all species
will be treated
with respect
and compassion.

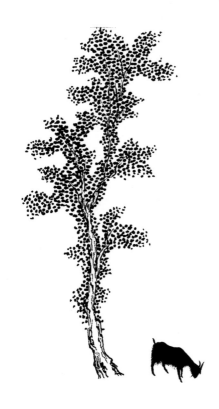

One who seeks understanding
of the meaning of life,
and insight
into the purpose
of creation,
finds beauty
within all beings—
no matter how foreign,
how unattractive,
or how different
such beings might be.

Such a seeker
is drawn to
the humble lifestyle
of a vegetarian.

Vegetarians live following the commandment—

Thou shall not kill.

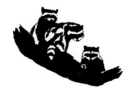

Those whose hearts go out
to all beings
who seek nothing more
than freedom
and a chance to live

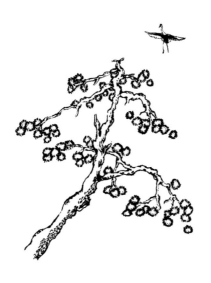

cannot help but become vegetarian.

Vegetarians value the words
of Khalil Gibran in *The Prophet* that

Life longs for itself.

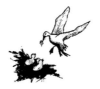

They strive to protect all who long to live.

Vegetarians easily forgo
their own pleasure
for the welfare
of other beings.

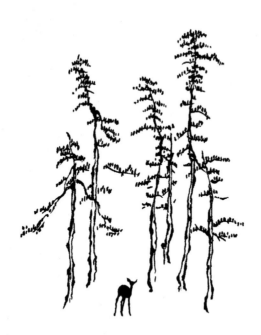

To vegetarians,
all life is sacred.

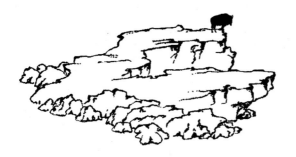

Vegetarians
recognize the vulnerability
and frailty
of all life.
They value the humble teaching—

Therefore, but for the grace of God go I.

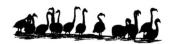

Vegetarians recognize

that each of us is just a humble being

in the perpetual flow of life

on this planet.

Vegetarians know that one's body
is merely a vehicle to transport one's soul.
Accordingly, they look beyond
the external appearance of all beings.

They value the soul of each.

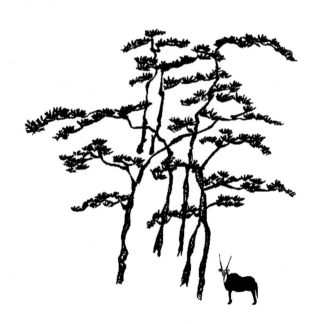

Vegetarians
feel joy
seeing birds
in flight.

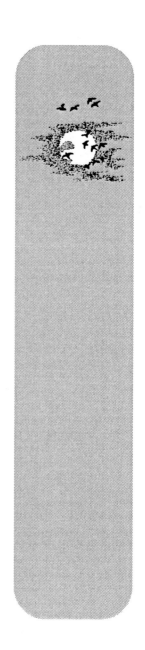

They send forth
blessings
of peace & joy
towards each
of them.

Those who cannot bear to inflict harm
on any innocent being—live as vegetarians.

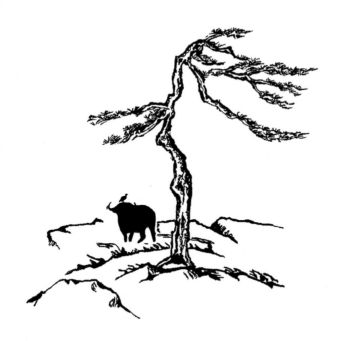

Those who recognize
that they can sustain their existence
without the consumption of flesh,
cannot bear to take life
from any being.

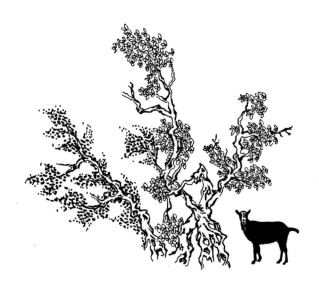

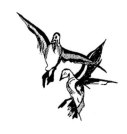

Vegetarians look forward to the day
when humankind seeks to create
a world
without bloodshed.

Vegetarians value the teachings of
Gautama Buddha, that

Wherever one encounters living beings,
one should feel towards them
as one feels
toward's one's own family.
Looking on each being
as one's child,
one will refrain from eating meat.

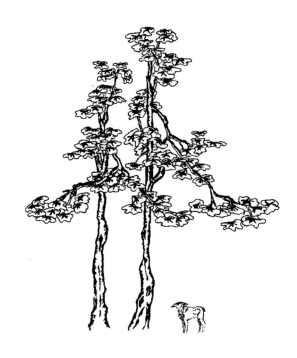

Those who feel humbled
by the miracle of creation

live as vegetarians.

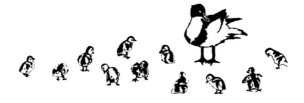

Vegetarians recognize that
one who lives without consuming flesh
is blessed—

blessed physically and spiritually.

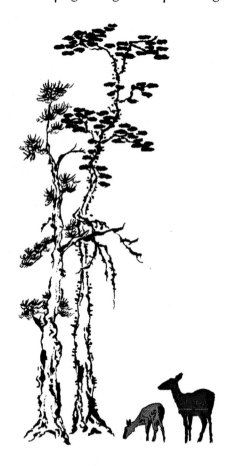

Vegetarians believe that only when
humankind acts
humane,
caring,
and justly
toward all beings—

will there be peace
on this planet.

Vegetarians believe that humankind
possesses the opportunity,
and the obligation,
to bestow dignity upon all beings.

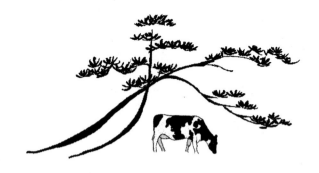

Those who recognize that consumption
of animal flesh involves the act of killing—

become vegetarian.

Vegetarians believe
that their refusal
to consume the flesh of other beings
is a strong act in support

of the cause of mercy.

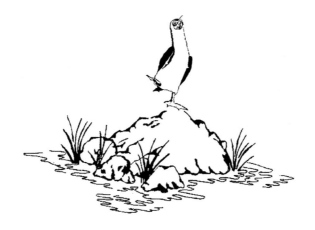

Vegetarians value the teachings of
Mahatma Gandhi,
that by consuming the flesh
of other beings—

We kill ourselves, our body and soul.

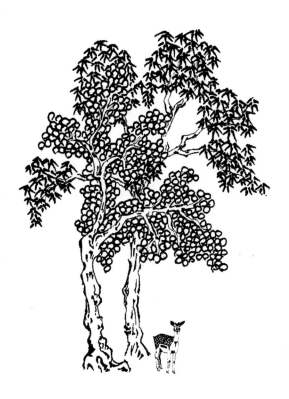

Vegetarians feel joy
seeing any being
safely and peacefully
enjoy life.

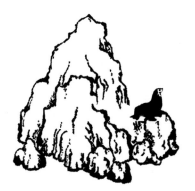

All vegetarians want
to live simply and humbly
without harming any other beings—

and they do.

Vegetarians feel fortunate
that they
have been given the
wisdom to
recognize
the value in all life.

They carry
this wisdom
with dignity
and humility.

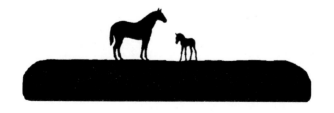

Vegetarians believe
that because a Higher Power
has given life to all beings,
only that Power
has the right
to reclaim such life.

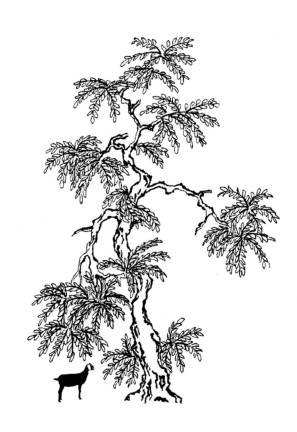

Vegetarians pray that all beings
may live out
their alloted lifespan.

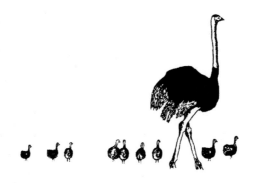

Vegetarians know
there is no need
to eat flesh.

They recognize they are
healthy,
satiated &
strong—
in body, mind and spirit—
without this.

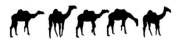

Vegetarians do not believe
that weaker beings
belong to them.

They believe that all beings
belong to themselves.

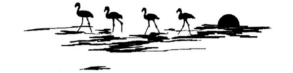

Vegetarians
look upon
all beings
with the soul
of a friend.

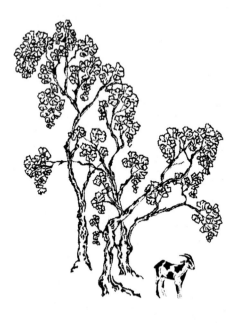

Vegetarians cannot bear to take the life
of any being
 whose eyes can look back
and plead for mercy.

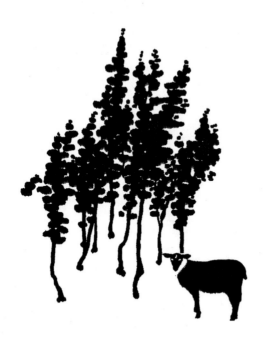

Vegetarians quietly
respect the values
of non-vegetarians.

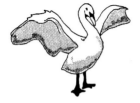

They recognize that
each individual
must follow
his or her own path.

Vegetarians seek to follow
all that is merciful
all that is gentle
all that is peaceful
all that is kind.

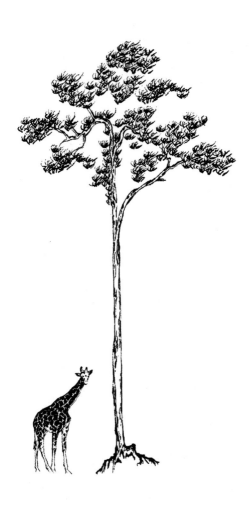

Vegetarians take no more
from this blessed planet
than they need.

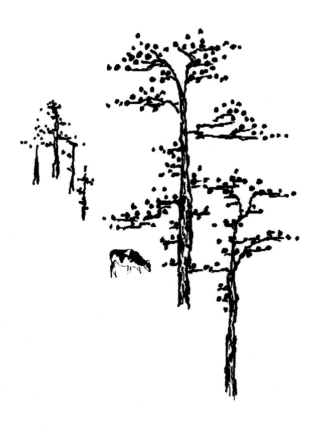

Vegetarians feel so sad
when they see any being harmed.
Hence,
they seek to live
without inflicting harm
on any of them.

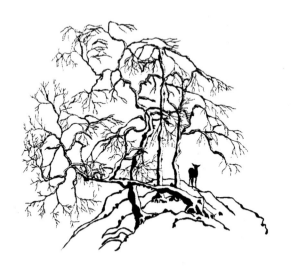

By not consuming flesh,
vegetarians have prevented
thousands and thousands
of innocent beings
from suffering.

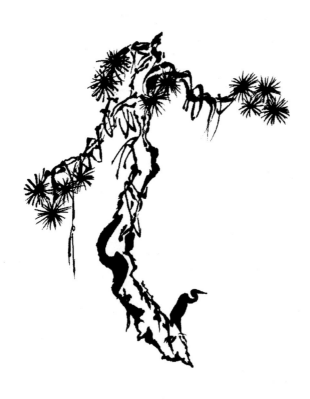

Vegetarians recognize
that life exists
at many different levels.
They respect
the value of life
within each.

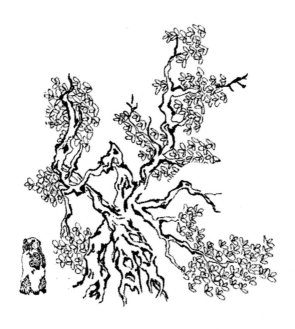

Vegetarians do not take it upon themselves
to judge which beings have a right to live
and which do not.
They seek to leave this decision
to a Higher Judge.

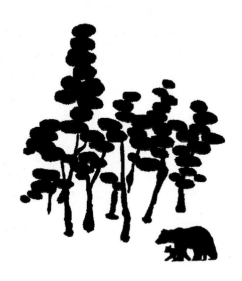

Vegetarians cannot help but be saddened
when the young of any species is harmed.

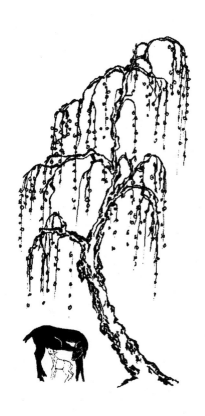

Vegetarians feel that the gentle cow
has harmed no one,
and that by harming her,
one harms all creation—
including oneself.

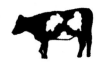

Vegetarians believe that all lives
are interconnected—
when one being suffers,
all suffer.

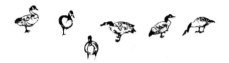

Vegetarians hope
their lives may become
examples
that kindle sparks of
enlightened compassion
in the souls of others.

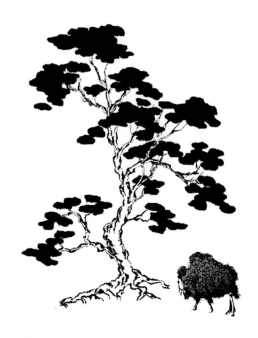

Vegetarians
feed
the
birds.

Vegetarians feel that before asking
God for mercy,
they, too, must show mercy
      to all others.

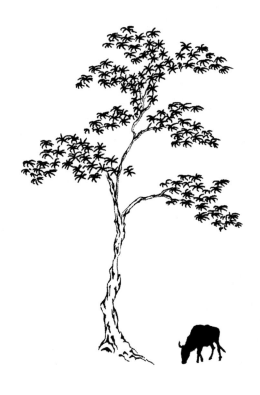

Vegetarians do not view
other species
as inferior.
They view
each and every species
as possessing
tremendous value.

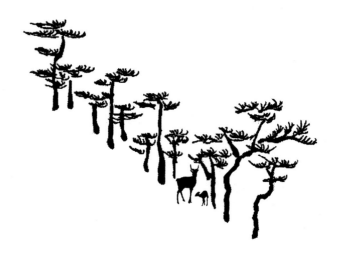

Although
compassionate
vegetarians
may
not
have
met
one
another,
they
know
there
are
others
out there
of
kindred
spirit.

Vegetarians look at
the humblest of beings
and remember—
    The first will be last
    and the last first.

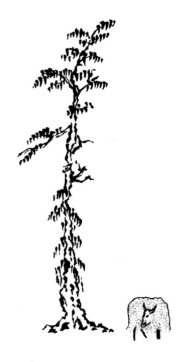

Compassionate vegetarians
have no doubts
that their diet
is healthy—

How could a diet
of compassion
not be?

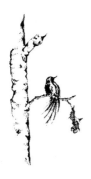

Vegetarians recognize
that throughout history,
there have been
countless other
compassionate vegetarians —

men and women with
integrity,
wisdom,
and kindness,
who have walked
quiet,
humble,
and peaceful
lifepaths—

just like theirs.

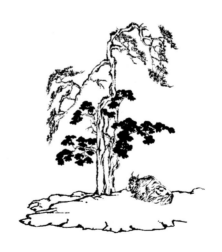

Vegetarians believe in the wisdom,

I may pass this way but once.
Let me show mercy, compassion,
and kindness to all.

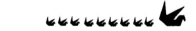

Printed in the United States
53743LVS00002B/229-231